COMPLETE GUIDE TO UNDERSTANDING LUMBAR DISCECTOMY

Essential Information On Surgical Techniques, Recovery, And Pain Management For Back Surgery Success

KLEIN HOYLE

Disclaimer

The content in this book is based on the author's expertise and comprehension of the topic. The author has no affiliation or link with any corporation, business, or person. This book is meant to give general information and educational material only, and it should not be interpreted as professional medical advice. Always seek the advice of a skilled healthcare expert if you have any queries about medical issues or treatments. The author and publisher expressly disclaim any responsibility resulting directly or indirectly from the use or use of the information included in this book.

ABOUT THIS BOOK

The "Complete Guide to Understanding Lumbar Discectomy" is a useful reference for both individuals and healthcare professionals navigating the complex world of spinal health. Beginning with an enlightening introduction in Chapter 1, the book delves into the substance of Lumbar Discectomy, demystifying its aim and demonstrating its importance. Readers will go on a journey that reveals the subtle relationship between surgical intervention and patient well-being, underlining the critical role of educated decision-making.

Chapter 2 dives into the complicated architecture of the spine, offering light on its multidimensional structure and the critical function of intervertebral discs. By explaining the importance of spinal alignment and the complicated network of nerves, the book establishes the groundwork for understanding the next chapters. Moving further, Chapter 3 delves deeply into the nuances of disc herniation, revealing its origins, symptoms, and significant influence on everyday life. Readers receive significant insights into the complexities of this illness thanks to a thorough examination, helping them to manage its obstacles with fortitude and knowledge.

Chapter 4 focuses on the key features of diagnosis, emphasizing the need for early detection and the many diagnostic techniques available. By precisely outlining common symptoms and differential diagnoses, the book provides readers with the skills they need to start on the road to successful treatment. As the trip proceeds, Chapter 5 provides a comprehensive overview of surgical preparation, stressing the need for pre-operative assessments, psychological preparedness, and informed consent.

The surgical process is meticulously explored in Chapter 6, which serves as the book's heart. Readers are taken through the technical details of different methods, anesthetic alternatives, and probable intraoperative problems, giving a thorough roadmap for both patients and healthcare professionals. Subsequent chapters explore the landscape of recovery, post-operative care, and long-term repercussions, providing a comprehensive view of the path to regained spine health.

Furthermore, in Chapter 9, the book discusses the intricacies of post-operative problems and the importance of lifestyle changes, equipping readers to face the difficulties of post-surgical life with fortitude and grace. The "Complete Guide to Understanding Lumbar Discectomy" is an invaluable companion for all people beginning on the road to spinal health and well-being, thanks to a careful balance of medical competence and caring instruction.

CHAPTER 1

Introduction To Lumbar Discectomy

What Is A Lumbar Discectomy?

Lumbar discectomy is a surgical operation used to treat discomfort caused by a herniated or bulging disc in the lower back (lumbar spine). This problem develops when the soft inner core of a spinal disc pushes through the strong outer layer, exerting pressure on adjacent nerves. To relieve symptoms such as leg discomfort, numbness, or weakness, the section of the disc pushing on the nerve is removed during surgery.

During the operation, the surgeon creates a tiny incision in the lower back and inserts specialized tools into the damaged disc. The herniated or bulging section of the disc is carefully removed, enabling the nerve to decompress and operate properly.

Who Needs A Lumbar Discectomy?

Lumbar discectomy is often advised for those who have not responded to non-surgical therapies such as physical therapy, medication, or steroid injections. Candidates for this operation often report acute or debilitating pain that interferes with their everyday activities and quality of life.

Common Indications For Lumbar Discectomy Are:

• Persistent discomfort or numbness down one or both legs.

• Experience muscle weakness or lack of feeling in legs or feet.

• Difficulty walking or standing for long periods owing to discomfort.

• Nerve compression may cause bladder/bowel dysfunction.

Before surgery, patients are subjected to a thorough assessment to confirm the diagnosis and evaluate if they are acceptable candidates for the treatment.

Purpose And Goals Of Surgery

The main purpose of a lumbar discectomy is to alleviate pressure on the spinal nerves produced by a herniated or bulging disc. The procedure seeks to reduce pain, numbness, and other symptoms associated with nerve compression by removing the section of the disc that impinges on the nerve.

In addition to discomfort alleviation, lumbar discectomy may assist improve mobility and function in those whose daily activities are hampered by back or leg pain. Patients may have greater strength and sensation in the damaged leg(s) when normal nerve function is restored, enabling them to resume activities that they were unable to undertake before the operation.

Overview Of The Treatment Process

The treatment procedure for lumbar discectomy often starts with a complete assessment by a spine specialist, which may include a physical examination, imaging examinations such as MRI or CT scans, and nerve conduction testing. Once a diagnosis has been established and all conservative therapy has been exhausted, surgery may be advised.

Patients go through pre-operative preparation before surgery, which may include blood tests, imaging exams, and conversations with the surgical team regarding the operation and what to anticipate during recovery.

On the day of surgery, patients are normally admitted to the hospital or surgical facility and given anesthesia to ensure they are comfortable and pain-free during the process. The surgeon then conducts a discectomy via a tiny incision in the lower back, using specialized equipment and methods to remove the herniated or bulging disc.

Following surgery, patients are carefully observed in the recovery area before being transported to a hospital room or released home, depending on the postoperative situation. Recovery time varies depending on the person and the degree of the operation, but most patients may return to mild activities within a few weeks and progressively raise their level of activity as instructed by their physician. Physical therapy and rehabilitation may be prescribed to improve healing and avoid future spinal issues.

Overall, lumbar discectomy is a well-proven and successful therapeutic option for those who suffer from pain and other symptoms caused by herniated or bulging discs in their lower back.

CHAPTER 2

Anatomy Of The Spine

Structure Of The Spine

The spine, or spinal column, is the body's major support component, providing both stability and motion. It consists of 33 vertebrae that are classified into five regions: cervical, thoracic, lumbar, sacral, and coccygeal. The lumbar spine, found in the lower back, is made up of five vertebrae numbered L1–L5. These vertebrae are bigger and stronger than those in other places because they carry the bulk of the body's weight.

Each vertebra has a distinct structure, which includes a body that bears weight, pedicles, and laminae that create the vertebral arch, and processes for muscle attachment.

Intervertebral discs sit between the vertebrae and function as shock absorbers while also allowing for flexibility.

Function Of The Intervertebral Discs

Intervertebral discs are important components of the spine that reside between neighboring vertebrae. They are made up of a strong outer layer called the annulus fibrosus and a gel-like inner core known as the nucleus pulposus. These discs provide many roles, including cushioning between vertebrae, facilitating movement, and preserving vertebral spacing.

During actions like walking, jogging, and lifting, the discs absorb shock and distribute pressure uniformly throughout the spine, protecting vertebrae and adjacent tissues from being damaged. Additionally, the discs improve spinal flexibility, allowing for bending, twisting, and other motions.

Spinal Alignment Is Really Crucial

Maintaining good spinal alignment is critical for overall health and wellness. When the spine is properly aligned, the vertebrae and discs are in their ideal locations, which relieves pressure on the muscles, ligaments, and nerves. Proper alignment also encourages proper posture, which may help avoid back discomfort and other musculoskeletal problems.

However, poor posture, injury, or degenerative disorders may all disturb spinal alignment, resulting in misalignments or abnormalities such as kyphosis, lordosis, or scoliosis. If not addressed, these problems may lead to discomfort, reduced movement, and other issues.

Role Of Nerves In The Spine

The spine has a complicated network of nerves that carry messages from the brain to the rest of the body. The vertebrae protect these nerves, known as the spinal cord, which stretch from the base of the brain to the lumbar spine.

Spinal nerves branch out from the spinal cord and leave the spinal column via tiny gaps between vertebrae known as intervertebral foramina. These nerves provide sensation and motor function to particular areas of the body, enabling movement, touch perception, and other critical activities.

In addition to spinal nerves, the spine contains the autonomic nervous system, which regulates involuntary body activities including heart rate, digestion, and breathing. Any disturbance or compression of the spine's nerves may cause symptoms such as pain, numbness, weakness, or loss of function, emphasizing the need to maintain spinal health and resolve any abnormalities as soon as possible.

CHAPTER 3

Understanding Disc Herniation

Causes Of Disc Herniation

Disc herniation, also known as slipping disc or ruptured disc, happens when the soft inner core of a spinal disc pushes through the thick outer covering. Understanding the causes of disc herniation is critical for comprehending how the problem presents itself and how it might be treated.

A frequent cause is age-related deterioration. As we age, our spinal discs lose water content and suppleness, leaving them more susceptible to herniation from routine motions or stresses. Furthermore, repeated tension or pressure on the spine from activities such as heavy lifting, poor lifting technique, or rapid twisting movements may all lead to disc herniation.

Poor posture, weight, and heredity all have an impact on spinal alignment and raise the risk of disc herniation.

Symptoms Associated With Herniated Discs

Recognizing the signs of a herniated disc is critical for timely diagnosis and treatment. Symptoms may vary based on the location and degree of the herniation, but frequent indicators include:

• Herniated discs may produce localized or radiating discomfort in the afflicted region. This discomfort may get greater with movement, coughing, or sneezing.

• Pressure on surrounding nerves might cause numbness, tingling, or weakening in certain body areas. For example, a herniated disc in the lower back might produce numbness or paralysis in the legs.

• Affected nerves may cause muscular weakness, making it difficult to execute certain motions or jobs.

• Disc herniation may alter reflexes, resulting in reduced or exaggerated reactions.

How Disc Herniation Impacts Mobility And Sensation

The effect of disc herniation on movement and sensation varies according to the degree and location of the herniation. In general, ruptured discs may impinge on nerves, resulting in discomfort, weakness, and sensory abnormalities that limit movement.

For example, a herniated disc in the lumbar spine (lower back) might compress the sciatic nerve, causing sciatica. Sciatica may produce shooting pain, numbness, and tingling that spreads from the lower back down the buttocks and into the legs, making it difficult to stand, walk, or sit comfortably.

Similarly, a herniated disc in the cervical spine (neck) may compress nerves that service the arms, hands, and upper torso.

This may cause discomfort, weakness, and numbness in the upper extremities, affecting fine motor abilities, grip strength, and general movement.

Effects Of Disc Herniation On Daily Life

The effects of disc herniation on everyday life may be severe, impacting many areas of work, leisure, and personal activities. Simple actions such as bending, lifting, or sitting for long periods may become uncomfortable or difficult, resulting in limited mobility and usefulness.

Furthermore, prolonged pain and discomfort caused by disc herniation may alter sleep patterns, reduce quality of life, and lead to mental distress such as worry or depression. Individuals with severe herniated discs may have trouble doing everyday tasks, resulting in diminished independence and dependency on others for support.

Overall, knowing the origins, symptoms, and consequences of disc herniation is critical for successfully treating the illness and enhancing the quality of life for individuals afflicted. Individuals who recognize the indications early and seek proper medical treatment and rehabilitation may reduce the effect of disc herniation on everyday activities and restore functioning and mobility.

CHAPTER 4

Symptoms And Diagnosis

Common Symptoms Of Lumbar Disc Herniation

Lumbar disc herniation may present in a variety of ways, often producing stiffness and pain in the lower back area. One of the most common symptoms is back discomfort that may extend down one or both legs. The herniated disc compresses the spinal nerves, causing sciatica. Patients may notice numbness, tingling, or weakness in the afflicted leg or foot. The degree of symptoms might range from slight discomfort to crippling pain that interferes with everyday activities.

In addition to sciatica, people with lumbar disc herniation may have muscular weakness or atrophy in their legs, especially if the nerve compression impairs motor function. This weakness may impair mobility and stability, making it difficult to walk or do regular chores. Furthermore, some people have abnormalities in bowel or bladder function, such as trouble urinating or regulating bowel motions, however, these symptoms are uncommon.

It is critical to detect these symptoms immediately and seek medical assistance if they continue or worsen over time. Early identification allows for prompt intervention and care, which may avoid subsequent issues and improve patient outcomes.

Diagnostic Testing And Imaging Techniques

Lumbar disc herniation is normally diagnosed using a combination of clinical examination, medical history assessment, and diagnostic imaging. During the first appointment, healthcare experts will ask about the patient's symptoms, such as the location, duration, and degree of pain, as well as any accompanying neurological symptoms.

Physical examination tools, such as the straight leg raising test and muscular strength evaluation, assist doctors in determining nerve function and identifying probable regions of compression or inflammation. Furthermore, imaging examinations such as X-rays, MRI (magnetic resonance imaging), and CT (computed tomography) scans give comprehensive visualization of the spinal structures, making it possible to diagnose disc herniation, nerve impingement, and other abnormalities.

MRI is especially useful for analyzing soft tissue features such as intervertebral discs and spinal nerves because it provides higher contrast and resolution than other imaging modalities. CT scans may be used to analyze bony structures and identify fractures or bone spurs that might cause nerve compression.

Differential Diagnosis For Back Pain

Given the wide range of illnesses that may cause back pain, physicians must employ a differential diagnostic to differentiate between lumbar disc herniation and other possible causes. Common differential diagnoses include muscular strain or sprain, facet joint dysfunction, spinal stenosis, spondylolisthesis, and vertebral fractures.

Clinical characteristics, imaging findings, and responses to conservative therapies may aid in distinguishing between these disorders. muscular strain, for example, is characterized by localized discomfort and muscular spasms, while facet joint dysfunction may cause pain that is aggravated by certain motions or postures. Spinal stenosis, which is defined by the narrowing of the spinal canal, often causes neurogenic claudication symptoms such as leg discomfort during walking.

Healthcare practitioners may make an accurate diagnosis and develop an appropriate treatment plan based on the patient's history, symptoms, and diagnostic results.

The Importance Of Early Detection

Early identification of lumbar disc herniation is critical for several reasons. First, it enables healthcare practitioners to undertake prompt therapies targeted at easing symptoms, lowering inflammation, and avoiding additional nerve injury. Conservative therapies such as physical therapy, medicines, and steroid injections may successfully relieve pain and improve function in many individuals, particularly when started early in the course of the illness.

Furthermore, early identification promotes patient education and self-management options, allowing people to actively engage in their treatment and make lifestyle changes that improve spine health. Healthcare practitioners may assist patients avoid recurring herniation by teaching them optimal body mechanics, ergonomics, and exercise strategies.

Furthermore, early diagnosis allows healthcare personnel to carefully follow patients for red flags or indicators of growing neurological impairments, which might indicate the necessity for surgical intervention. If conservative therapies do not give substantial relief or there is evidence of considerable nerve compression, a lumbar discectomy may be considered to decompress the afflicted nerves and relieve symptoms.

Overall, early identification of lumbar disc herniation enables patients and healthcare professionals to adopt timely treatments, maximize treatment results, and improve the quality of life for people with this illness.

CHAPTER 5

Preparing For Surgery

Pre-Operative Assessments And Screenings

Before having lumbar discectomy surgery, patients will normally go through various pre-operative exams and screenings to ensure they are physically and emotionally prepared. These assessments are critical in recognizing any possible hazards or issues that may occur during or after surgery.

A comprehensive medical history review is one of the first elements in the preoperative procedure. This requires the patient to provide extensive information on their prior and present medical problems, medicines, allergies, and any previous procedures. This information assists the surgical team in understanding the patient's general health state and identifying any possible risks to the operation or recovery process.

In addition to a medical history review, patients will have a physical assessment. During this assessment, the surgeon will evaluate the patient's general health, including range of motion, strength, and feeling in the afflicted region. This allows the surgeon to identify the amount of disc herniation and any other spinal abnormalities that may exist.

Depending on the patient's medical history and physical examination results, further pre-operative testing may be required. These screenings may include blood tests, imaging examinations such as X-rays or MRI scans, and electrocardiograms (ECGs) to monitor heart function. These tests aid in detecting any underlying medical issues that may need to be treated before surgery.

Overall, pre-operative examinations and screenings are critical to the safety and efficacy of lumbar discectomy surgery. By carefully analyzing the patient's health state and identifying any possible risks or consequences, the surgical team may create a specific treatment plan that matches the patient's requirements while increasing the likelihood of a positive result.

Medications And Lifestyle Changes Before Surgery

Patients preparing for lumbar discectomy surgery may need to take medication and lifestyle changes to improve their health and limit the risk of problems during and after the treatment. These changes are usually indicated by the surgical team and may differ based on the patient's medical history and current health state.

Blood-thinning drugs, such as aspirin or warfarin, are often discontinued before surgery. These drugs might raise the risk of severe bleeding during surgery, thus patients are typically advised to discontinue them several days before the operation. However, patients must strictly adhere to their surgeon's recommendations and not discontinue any drugs without first talking with their healthcare practitioner.

In addition to medication modifications, patients may be recommended to adopt lifestyle changes to enhance their general health and lower their chance of surgical complications. This may involve stopping smoking, decreasing weight if needed, and increasing physical exercise. These lifestyle changes may assist enhance the body's capacity to mend after surgery, increasing the overall success percentage of the treatment.

Furthermore, patients may be advised to avoid activities or behaviors that may aggravate their spinal condition or raise the risk of complications. Patients may be advised to avoid heavy lifting, bending, or twisting actions, which may strain the spine and exacerbate symptoms.

Overall, drugs and lifestyle changes before lumbar discectomy surgery are intended to improve the patient's health and lower the chance of problems. Patients may ensure a good result for the treatment by adhering to the surgical team's instructions and making required modifications to their pharmaceutical regimen and lifestyle habits.

Psychological Preparation For Surgery

Preparing for lumbar discectomy surgery requires both physical and psychological fitness. It is normal for patients to be apprehensive or concerned about having surgery, but there are actions they can take to help control these feelings and feel more confident and peaceful in the run-up to the treatment.

Education is a key component of psychological preparedness. Patients should learn about the operation and what to anticipate before, during, and after surgery. This may assist in relieving worries and doubts by offering a better grasp of the procedure and what will occur at each step.

Relaxation and stress-reduction strategies are another effective psychological preparation tool. This might involve deep breathing techniques, meditation, yoga, or engaging in enjoyable and relaxing hobbies. Patients who include these activities in their regular routines might help soothe their anxiety and develop a feeling of well-being in the run-up to surgery.

Patients may also benefit from seeking assistance from friends, family members, or support groups who have had comparable surgeries. Talking to people who have gone through similar experiences may bring comfort, practical guidance, and a feeling of community and understanding.

Finally, open contact with the surgical team is essential for psychological preparedness. Patients should feel free to ask questions, voice concerns, and share any thoughts or anxiety they may have regarding the procedure. The surgical team may provide patients with information, advice, and support to make them feel more confident and prepared for the treatment.

By addressing psychological variables and taking proactive actions to control stress and anxiety, patients may help guarantee a smoother and more pleasant experience leading up to lumbar discectomy surgery. With the proper mentality and support system in place, patients may approach the surgery with confidence and excitement.

Discussion With The Surgical Team And Informed Consent

Before having lumbar discectomy surgery, patients should have a detailed conversation with their surgical team to ensure they thoroughly understand the operation, possible risks and advantages, and what to anticipate throughout the recovery period. This talk is a critical step in the informed consent process, ensuring that patients make well-informed healthcare choices.

Patients should be able to ask the surgical team any questions they may have concerning the procedure during the consultation. This might include inquiries regarding the surgical approach, anticipated results, possible risks, and alternative treatment choices. The surgical team should respond to these questions clearly and completely, as well as any extra information pertinent to the patient's situation.

In addition to discussing the treatment, the surgical team will analyze the patient's medical history and conduct a physical examination to determine their general health and readiness for surgery. This ensures that the patient is a suitable candidate for lumbar discectomy and that any possible risks or consequences are recognized and addressed before surgery.

Once all of the patient's questions have been addressed and they are satisfied with the information presented, they will be asked to provide informed permission for the procedure. Informed consent indicates that the patient is aware of the nature of the operation, as well as the possible risks, advantages, and alternatives, and willingly agrees to have the surgery.

Informed consent is not just a legal need, but also an ethical one, since it ensures that patients are actively engaged in their healthcare choices. Patients who engage in open and honest talks with their surgical team and provide informed consent might feel more secure and empowered as they prepare for lumbar discectomy surgery.

CHAPTER 6

Surgical Procedures

Types Of Lumbar Discectomy Techniques

Lumbar discectomy is a surgical operation used to treat discomfort caused by a herniated or ruptured disc in the lower back. Surgeons employ a variety of ways to accomplish this treatment, each with its own set of benefits and drawbacks.

Microdiscectomy

Microdiscectomy is one of the most popular procedures for lumbar discectomy. In this minimally invasive procedure, the surgeon creates a tiny incision around the damaged disc and removes the herniated section using sophisticated devices, including a microscope. Microdiscectomy has the benefit of allowing for fewer incisions, less tissue damage, and faster recovery periods than typical open surgery.

Endoscopic discectomy

Endoscopic discectomy is another minimally invasive procedure that uses a small camera called an endoscope to see into the spine. With this method, the surgeon inserts the endoscope via a small incision and removes the herniated disc material with small tools guided by the camera. Endoscopic discectomy has the benefit of smaller incisions and perhaps quicker recovery periods than microdiscectomy.

Open discectomy

Open discectomy is the conventional surgical method for lumbar discectomy. This approach involves the physician making a wider incision over the afflicted disc and removing the herniated section of the disc using surgical instruments. While open discectomy may take longer to recover and cause more postoperative discomfort than minimally invasive procedures, it may be essential in circumstances when the herniation is very big or complicated.

Anesthesia is essential for assuring patient comfort and safety during lumbar discectomy surgery. There are numerous choices available, depending on the patient's health and the surgeon's preferences.

General anesthesia

General anesthesia is giving the patient drugs to cause a brief loss of consciousness, enabling them to remain uninformed and pain-free during the treatment. During lumbar discectomy surgery, the patient is intubated to ensure a clean airway and an anesthesiologist or nurse anesthetist monitors vital signs constantly.

Regional Anesthesia

Regional anesthesia is injecting drugs near the nerves that feed the surgical area to numb it and suppress pain signals. One frequent form of regional anesthetic used for lumbar discectomy is spinal anesthesia, which involves injecting drugs into the spinal fluid to numb the bottom part of the body. Another alternative is epidural anesthesia, which involves injecting medicine into the epidural area around the spinal cord.

Local anesthesia

Local anesthetic is injecting medicine directly into the skin and tissues around the surgical site to numb it and block pain signals. While local anesthetic alone may not offer enough pain relief for lumbar discectomy surgery, it is sometimes combined with sedation or other types of anesthesia to improve patient comfort.

A Step-By-Step Breakdown Of The Surgical Procedure

Preoperative preparation

Before surgery, the patient is placed on the operating table and his or her vital signs are checked. The surgical team prepares the surgery site by cleaning it and covering it with sterile drapes to provide a sterile field.

Incision

The surgeon creates a tiny incision near the damaged disc, usually less than an inch long. The incision may be done vertically or horizontally, depending on the surgeon's discretion and the position of the hernia.

Access to the spine

To get access to the damaged disc, the surgeon delicately separates the muscles and soft tissues around the spine using specialist devices. In minimally invasive procedures such as microdiscectomy or endoscopic discectomy, the tissues are dilated rather than cut through.

Removal of Disc Material

Once the surgeon has gained access to the herniated disc, they will use surgical instruments to remove the section of the disc that is pushing on the nerves.

This might include cutting away the protruding disc material or suctioning it out using a vacuum-like apparatus.

Closure

After the disc material is removed, the surgeon gently heals the incision with sutures or surgical staples. In rare circumstances, a tiny drain may be inserted near the incision to collect excess fluid or blood.

Potential Intraoperative Complications

While lumbar discectomy is typically regarded as safe, several risks may develop during the surgical treatment. The complications include:

Nerve injury

During surgery, there is a danger of damaging the nerves that surround the spine, which may cause weakness, numbness, and other neurological abnormalities.

The surgeon makes great effort to reduce this danger by using specialized tools and methods.

Bleeding

Bleeding is a possible side effect of any surgical surgery, including lumbar discectomy. While small bleeding may usually be managed with cauterization or pressure, severe bleeding may need further procedures such as blood transfusion or surgical investigation.

Infection

Infection is a problem after every surgical surgery, and the spine is no exception. The surgical team makes efforts to reduce the risk of infection, such as utilizing sterile methods and giving antibiotics before and after the procedure.

Dural Tear

A dural tear happens when the outermost layer of the spinal cord is accidentally ruptured during surgery. While dural rips are uncommon, they may result in consequences such as cerebrospinal fluid leaks or infection. The surgeon may patch the rip during surgery or take extra precautions to avoid problems.

Recurrence of symptoms

In certain circumstances, lumbar disc herniation symptoms may reappear after surgery, either because the disc material was not completely removed or because additional disc herniations formed. The surgeon regularly monitors the patient's symptoms and may propose further treatments as needed.

CHAPTER 7

Recovery Process

Immediate Postoperative Care

Following lumbar discectomy surgery, urgent post-operative care is critical to ensure a successful healing phase. Once the operation is done, the patient is usually sent to a recovery area where they are carefully followed by medical personnel. To guarantee stability, the patient's vital signs are continuously monitored, including blood pressure, heart rate, and respiration. Pain management is also used to make the patient comfortable throughout the first recovery phase.

One of the key purposes of initial post-operative care is to look for any indicators of problems that may develop after surgery. This includes keeping an eye out for excessive bleeding, infection, or anesthesia-related complications.

The surgical site is checked frequently for any symptoms of redness, swelling, or drainage, which might signal infection. The medical team responds quickly to any concerns or changes in the patient's state to prevent issues from progressing.

In addition, the patient may be given particular instructions for wound care and activity limitations in the early postoperative period. This may involve keeping the surgical incision clean and dry, avoiding movements or postures that may strain the surgical site, and adhering to any recommended drug regimes.

Physiotherapy And Rehabilitation Exercises

Physical therapy and rehabilitation activities are essential in the healing process after lumbar discectomy surgery. While surgery treats the underlying cause of pain or suffering, physical therapy works to restore strength, flexibility, and function to the afflicted region.

Physical therapy in the early phases of rehabilitation may concentrate on mild motions and exercises to reduce pain and inflammation, improve range of motion, and avoid stiffness. This might include activities like mild stretching, low-impact exercises, and mobility exercises to assist the patient gradually restore strength and function.

As the patient's rehabilitation proceeds, physical therapy activities may become more difficult and focus on particular objectives, such as developing core strength, stability, and posture. The physical therapist collaborates closely with the patient to create a customized workout program based on their specific requirements and skills.

Consistency and commitment to the physical therapy plan are critical for excellent results after lumbar discectomy surgery. Patients are often advised to do their prescribed exercises at home regularly in addition to their supervised treatment sessions to maximize their healing potential.

Gradual Resumption Of Everyday Activities

Following lumbar discectomy surgery, patients should gradually resume their normal activities in a safe and regulated way. While it is natural to want to resume regular activities as soon as possible, it is important to listen to your body and avoid pushing yourself too hard, too soon.

During the recuperation phase, patients may suffer varied degrees of pain, discomfort, and exhaustion, limiting their ability to conduct specific tasks. It is critical to pace oneself and gradually raise activity levels as tolerated while being cognizant of any limits or precautions imposed by the medical team.

The timing for returning to various activities will differ based on the patient's recovery status and the type of operation. Some patients may be able to resume modest activities, such as walking or light housework, within a few days or weeks after surgery, while others may need a longer time to heal before returning to more demanding activities.

Patients need to talk honestly with their healthcare professionals about their progress and any difficulties they may be facing throughout their rehabilitation. This enables the medical team to provide advice and assistance as required to ensure a safe and successful return to normal activities.

Monitoring For Indicators Of Problems

Throughout the healing process, keep a watchful eye out for any indicators of problems that may emerge as a result of lumbar discectomy surgery. While problems are uncommon, they may occur and may need immediate medical intervention to avoid more difficulties or long-term repercussions.

Complications after lumbar discectomy surgery may include increased pain or discomfort, swelling, redness, or discharge at the surgical site, fever, chills, or other indicators of infection, numbness or weakness in the legs or feet, and problems with bladder or bowel function.

Patients are usually given precise advice on what signs and symptoms to look for and when to seek medical help if they appear. It is critical to properly follow these recommendations and do not hesitate to call the medical staff if any problems emerge.

In rare circumstances, further imaging scans or tests may be required to assess any possible problems. Early diagnosis and action are critical for successfully treating problems and fostering a full recovery after lumbar discectomy surgery.

CHAPTER 8

Postoperative Care

Wound Treatment And Incision Management

Proper wound care and incision control are critical components of postoperative care after a lumbar discectomy. Your surgeon will give you specific recommendations based on your unique condition, but there are some broad rules to follow.

First and foremost, keep the incision site clean and dry. You may be asked to gently clean the area with light soap and water, taking care not to scrape or aggravate the incision. Pat the area dry with a clean cloth or let it air dry. Avoid immersing the incision in water until your surgeon gives the go-ahead, which is usually around two weeks following surgery.

Monitoring for symptoms of infection is also an important part of wound care. Keep a lookout for increasing redness, swelling, warmth, or drainage at the incision site. If you have any of these symptoms or develop a fever, call your healthcare practitioner right away, since they may suggest an infection that needs emergency treatment.

It is also critical to follow any special instructions issued by your surgeon about dressing changes, topical ointments, or antibiotics. Some surgeons may advise keeping the wound covered with a sterile covering for a particular amount of time to encourage healing and limit the risk of infection.

Pain Management Strategies

Pain management is a major issue after a lumbar discectomy, however, there are numerous ways to reduce pain and promote recovery.

To treat postoperative pain, your surgeon may prescribe pain medication. It is important to take these drugs exactly as prescribed and to talk with your doctor if you suffer insufficient pain relief or any serious side effects.

In addition to medicine, non-pharmacological pain management strategies might be beneficial. These may include cold or heat treatment, light stretching and strengthening exercises, and relaxation methods like deep breathing or guided visualization.

Physical therapy may also aid in pain management and healing. Your surgeon may suggest that you begin a physical therapy program to gradually restore strength, flexibility, and function to the damaged region.

Guidelines For Resumed Work And Physical Activities

Returning to work and physical activity after a lumbar discectomy requires careful thought and advice from your healthcare team. It is critical to follow any particular recommendations issued by your surgeon and gradually return to your usual routine.

In general, you may need to take some time off from work to enable your body to recuperate fully. Your surgeon will advise you on when it is safe to return to work, depending on the nature of your profession and the physical demands it requires.

When it comes to physical activities, it is important to begin cautiously and gradually raise the intensity over time. Avoid lifting heavy things or indulging in intense activities until your surgeon gives you the go-ahead, which is usually six to eight weeks after surgery.

Listen to your body and be aware of any discomfort or pain when exercising. If you notice any new or worsening symptoms, stop what you're doing and visit your doctor.

Follow-Up Appointments And Monitoring

Regular follow-up meetings with your surgeon are necessary to evaluate your progress and handle any concerns or issues that may occur.

During these sessions, your surgeon will evaluate your healing process, keep an eye out for symptoms of infection or other problems, and make any necessary adjustments to your treatment plan. They may also prescribe imaging tests, such as X-rays or MRIs, to assess the surgery site and ensure adequate recovery.

In addition to follow-up consultations with your surgeon, you may be referred to additional healthcare experts, such as physical therapists or pain management specialists, to assist with your rehabilitation.

Attend all planned follow-up visits and talk honestly with your healthcare provider if you have any questions or concerns. You may increase your chances of success after lumbar discectomy surgery by being proactive and involved in your recovery process.

CHAPTER 9

Complications And Risks

Common Complications Of Lumbar Discectomy

While lumbar discectomy is typically considered safe and successful, there are certain risks and problems to consider. Infection is a frequent complication. Despite precautions, the surgical site may get infected, resulting in symptoms such as increased pain, edema, redness, and fever. The infection needs immediate medical treatment and may involve antibiotics or, in extreme circumstances, further surgical surgery to resolve.

Nerve injury is yet another potential consequence. While the operation is meant to alleviate pressure on nerves injured by a herniated disc, there is a danger of inadvertent nerve injury during the process. This may cause symptoms such as numbness, weakness, or sensory alterations. Nerve injury is usually transient and recovers on its own over time, but any new or worsening symptoms should be properly monitored.

Additionally, there is a danger of blood clots developing in the legs or lungs (deep vein thrombosis or pulmonary embolism) after lumbar discectomy. These clots may be deadly if they reach essential organs, thus precautions such as early mobilization, compression stockings, and blood-thinning drugs may be advised.

Other potential issues are:

• Excessive bleeding during or after surgery may necessitate transfusion or surgical intervention.

• During surgery, the dura mater, the spinal cord's protective covering, might rip accidentally, causing cerebrospinal fluid leaking and infection risk.

• Recurrent disc herniation: Surgery may not always resolve a herniated disc, necessitating further intervention.

• Anesthesia-related complications may arise after lumbar discectomy, including allergic responses, respiratory difficulties, and cardiovascular concerns.

While these problems are conceivable, it is important to realize that the vast majority of lumbar discectomy operations are successful and provide patients with relief from symptoms. However, being aware of potential hazards and responding to them quickly may help ensure the best possible results.

Risk Factors That Can Increase Complications

Several variables may raise the risk of problems after lumbar discectomy. This includes:

• Obesity may make surgery more difficult and raise the risk of complications including infection, blood clots, and poor wound healing.

• Tobacco smoking may affect circulation and delay wound healing, leading to an increased risk of infection and post-operative problems.

• Poorly managed diabetes may reduce the body's capacity to heal wounds and fight infections, raising the risk of surgical complications.

• Age: Older persons may have underlying health issues or lower physiological reserves, increasing the risk of complications during and after surgery.

• Patients who have had prior spine surgery may have scar tissue or changed anatomy, complicating future treatments.

• Certain medical diseases, including cardiovascular illness, respiratory disorders, and autoimmune conditions, might increase the risk of complications during surgery and recovery.

Before having a lumbar discectomy, individuals must consult with their healthcare professional about their medical history and potential risks. Identifying and treating possible risk factors may assist in reducing the number of complications and enhance surgical results.

Strategies To Prevent Complications

While difficulties are not always completely avoidable, numerous methods might help lower the likelihood of adverse events after lumbar discectomy:

• Optimizing patients' health before surgery, especially addressing chronic medical disorders like diabetes or hypertension, may lower the chance of complications.

• Antibiotic prophylaxis helps prevent surgical site infections.

• Prophylaxis for deep vein thrombosis (DVT) includes early mobilization, compression stockings, and blood-thinning drugs to lower the risk of blood clots.

• Precise surgical technique, including minimal tissue stress, may lower the likelihood of consequences such as nerve injury and dural tears.

• Close monitoring of patients after surgery helps discover and treat issues including infection or neurological impairments.

• Educating patients about possible problems, warning signals, and postoperative care may help them take an active part in their recovery and seek medical assistance as required.

Healthcare practitioners may assist patients having lumbar discectomy to avoid problems and improve their results by taking these preventative practices.

When To Seek Medical Attention For Post-Operative Issues

While some pain and movement limits are anticipated after a lumbar discectomy, several problems need immediate medical attention:

• Pain that persists or worsens despite medicine or rest.

• Symptoms of infection may include fever, chills, redness, edema, or discharge at the surgical site.

• Experiencing new or worsening neurological symptoms, including weakness, numbness, or changes in bowel or bladder function.

• Difficulty breathing or chest discomfort might suggest a pulmonary embolism.

• Excessive bleeding or drainage at the surgical site.

If patients have any of these symptoms after having a lumbar discectomy, they should contact their healthcare physician right once. Early action may assist to avoid difficulties and get the best potential result.

CHAPTER 10

Lifestyle Following Lumbar Discectomy

Long-Term Impact Of Surgery On Mobility And Functionality

Lumbar discectomy surgery is designed to relieve pain and enhance mobility by removing herniated disc material that may be pushing on nerves in the spine. While the immediate post-operative phase may be uncomfortable and limiting while the body recovers, many patients will see considerable gains in mobility and functioning as a result of the operation in the long run.

Following surgery, patients often report improvement from problems that had previously limited their movement, such as limb discomfort, numbness, or paralysis. As the healing process progresses, patients may recover strength and flexibility in the damaged region.

Physical therapy and rehabilitation programs customized to each patient's specific requirements may help improve mobility and function over time.

However, patients must recognize that the effectiveness of lumbar discectomy surgery in recovering mobility and functioning varies depending on several circumstances, including the amount of disc herniation, the patient's general health, and adherence to post-operative care protocols. Some individuals may continue to endure symptoms or limits following surgery, whilst others may fully recover to their pre-injury level of activity.

Recommendations To Maintain Spinal Health

Maintaining spinal health is critical for avoiding future problems and improving the outcome of lumbar discectomy surgery. Patients may take several proactive activities to improve spinal health and limit the chance of recurrence or new injuries:

1. Regular Exercise: Low-impact activities like walking, swimming, or yoga may help strengthen and stretch the muscles that support the spine. It is critical to work with a healthcare practitioner or physical therapist to create a safe and effective fitness program that is customized to your specific requirements and limits.

2. Proper Body Mechanics: Maintaining appropriate posture and lifting methods may assist lessen pressure on the spine and lower the chance of injury. Avoiding lengthy periods of sitting or standing in the same posture, as well as adopting ergonomic furniture or equipment wherever feasible, may all help with spinal health.

3. Healthy Lifestyle Choices: Maintaining a healthy weight, eating a balanced diet rich in nutrients that promote bone health, and quitting smoking may all improve spine health and general well-being. Smoking, in particular, may hinder the body's capacity to recover, raising the chance of problems after surgery.

4. Regular Check-ups: Routine visits to healthcare professionals for check-ups and screenings may help spot possible problems early and give appropriate intervention if necessary. Patients should adhere to their surgeon's advice for follow-up treatment and monitoring after lumbar discectomy surgery.

Coping Strategies For Managing Chronic Pain (If Present)

While many patients enjoy great pain relief after lumbar discectomy surgery, others may continue to endure chronic pain or discomfort as a result of underlying spinal problems or other causes. Coping methods may assist people in managing chronic pain and enhancing their quality of life:

1. Pain Management methods: Learning and practicing relaxation methods like deep breathing, meditation, and guided imagery may help decrease tension and pain.

Additionally, over-the-counter or prescription drugs recommended by a healthcare physician may aid with pain management.

2. Physical Therapy: Participating in a systematic physical therapy program may assist in increasing strength, flexibility, and range of motion, resulting in less discomfort and improved functional skills. A physical therapist may provide customized exercises and approaches to treat particular pain patterns and restrictions.

3. Mind-Body Approaches: Cognitive-behavioral therapy (CBT) and biofeedback are two techniques that may help patients build coping skills and control the psychological effects of chronic pain. These tactics are aimed at modifying negative thinking patterns, enhancing coping skills, and encouraging relaxation.

4. Support Networks: Connecting with people who have had similar issues may give emotional support as well as practical assistance for chronic pain management.

Support groups, whether in person or online, may provide a feeling of connection and understanding.

The Significance Of Regular Follow-Up Care And Monitoring

Following lumbar discectomy surgery, ongoing follow-up care and monitoring are required to achieve optimum results and discover any possible problems early. Patients should follow their surgeon's suggested follow-up program, which might include:

1. **Post-operative Visits:** Appointments with the surgeon or healthcare practitioner are scheduled to monitor the healing process, evaluate mobility and function, and address any concerns or symptoms that may occur.

2. **Imaging Studies:** Follow-up imaging tests, such as X-rays or MRI scans, may be requested to review the surgery site and look for evidence of recurrence, complications, or new spinal concerns.

3. Physical Therapy: Attending physical therapy sessions as prescribed will aid in continued healing, treat any residual limits or symptoms, and maintain long-term spine health.

4. Medication Management: If drugs were recommended to treat pain or other conditions, follow-up appointments let you assess their efficacy, change doses as needed, and address any side effects or concerns.

5. Lifestyle Recommendations: Healthcare practitioners may advise patients on lifestyle changes, exercise programs, and ergonomic improvements that are customized to their specific circumstances to enhance spine health and avoid future problems.

Patients who prioritize frequent follow-up treatment and monitoring may collaborate with their healthcare team to improve their recovery, manage any residual difficulties, and preserve long-term spine health and function.

Conclusion

In conclusion, a lumbar discectomy is a surgical treatment performed to treat pain and other symptoms caused by a herniated disc in the lower back. Throughout this thorough guide, we have looked at all elements of lumbar discectomy, from indications and preparation to surgical procedures and post-operative care.

First, we spoke about the structure of the lumbar spine and the function of intervertebral discs, focusing on how a herniated disc may cause nerve compression and accompanying symptoms like pain, numbness, and weakness. Understanding the underlying pathology is critical in selecting the best treatment option, and for many patients with chronic symptoms, a lumbar discectomy may provide considerable relief.

We then moved on to the assessment procedure, which included a full medical history, physical examination, and diagnostic imaging investigations including MRIs and CT scans. These examinations assist in confirming the diagnosis and determine the exact position and extent of the disc herniation, which guides the surgical strategy.

The guide next went over the different surgical methods used in lumbar discectomy, including classic open surgery and less invasive treatments like microdiscectomy. Each procedure has benefits and disadvantages, and the decision is based on criteria such as the patient's anatomy, the degree of symptoms, and the surgeon's experience.

We also spoke about the dangers and problems of lumbar discectomy, such as infection, nerve injury, and recurrent disc herniation. While the dangers are modest, people should be aware of them and make educated decisions with their healthcare professionals.

Post-operative care and rehabilitation are critical components of a full recovery following lumbar discectomy. We emphasized the need to follow the surgeon's recommendations for activity limits, pain management, and physical therapy to improve results and reduce the risk of complications.

Finally, we underlined the need for long-term treatment techniques, such as lifestyle changes, ergonomic principles, and regular exercise, in preventing disc herniation and maintaining spinal health.

Lumbar discectomy is an effective therapeutic option for those who are suffering from severe symptoms caused by a herniated disc in their lower back. We hope that by offering a full knowledge of this surgical treatment, patients and healthcare providers will be able to make educated choices and achieve the best possible results in the management of lumbar disc herniation.

THE END